My Keto Cookbook

An Unmissable Recipe Collection

for Your Low-Carb Daily Meals

Kimberly Wood

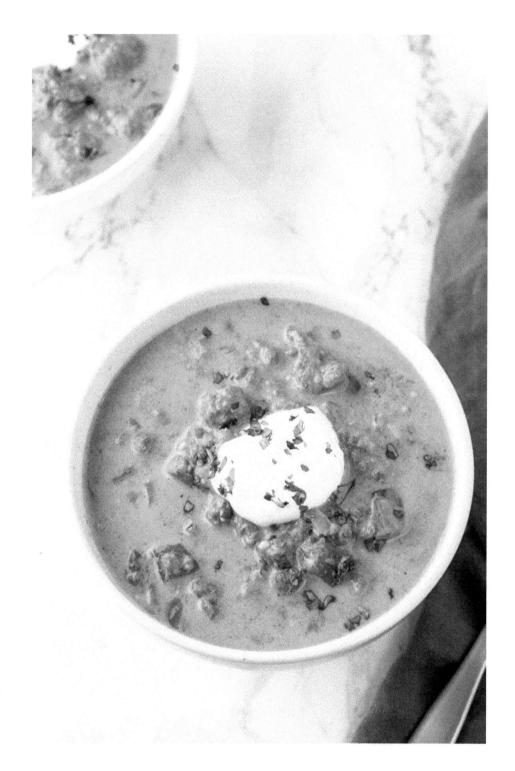

Table of Contents

POULTRY

Lemon-Rosemary Roasted Cornish Hens

Macros: Fat 66% | Protein 30% | Carbs 4%

Prep time: 10 minutes | Cook time: 55 minutes | Serves 4

If you are only ever going to really master a single recipe, let it be this one! It's really simple. If you can cook chicken, you can cook cornish game hen.

This Cornish Game Hen Recipe is perfect for any occasion! The bright flavors of the lemon and rosemary will have everyone on the planet go crazy for having it and still wanting more.

- 4 Cornish game hen
- Salt and freshly ground black pepper, to taste
- 3 tablespoons olive oil
- 4 sprigs fresh rosemary, plus 4 more sprigs for garnish
- 2 teaspoons paprika
- 1 lemon, quartered
- 24 cloves garlic
- ⅓ cup low-sodium chicken broth
- ⅓ cup dry white wine

Preheat the oven to 450°F (235°C).

Make the marinade: In a small bowl, stir together the salt, pepper, 2 tablespoons of olive oil, rosemary, and paprika. Set aside.

Clean and dry each hen. Squeeze the lemon juice inside the cavity and on the surface of each hen. Place 1 sprig of rosemary and 1 lemon wedge inside each hen. Evenly rub each hen with the marinade until well coated.

Place hens in a large roasting dish (at least an inch apart) and arrange garlic cloves around hens. (A bit of space between each hen leads to even browning and crispy skin.)

Place the roasting dish in the preheated oven and roast for about 25 minutes.

Reduce the oven temperature to 350°F (180°C).

Combine the remaining olive oil, chicken broth, and wine in a mixing bowl. Pour the mixture over hens and continue roasting for 25 minutes, or until hens are a deep golden color and reach at least 165°F (74°C) on a meat thermometer.

Remove the hens from the oven to a plate. Pour any remaining juices and garlic cloves to a medium saucepan. Cover the hens with aluminum foil to keep warm.

Boil the left juices and garlic cloves in the saucepan for 6 minutes until the liquid thickens to a sauce consistency.

Cut each hen half lengthwise into slices and place on serving plates. Pour the sauce and garlic cloves over them. Garnish with rosemary sprigs on top before serving.

STORAGE: Store in an airtight container in the fridge for up to 4 days or in the freezer for up to 1 month.

REHEAT: Microwave, covered, until the desired temperature is reached or reheat in a frying pan or air fryer / instant pot, covered, on medium.

SERVE IT WITH: To make this a complete meal, serve these hens alongside some mushrooms cooked in the hen juices.

PER SERVING

calories: 796 | fat: 58.3g | total carbs: 10.5g | fiber: 2.5g | protein: 59.8g

Grilled Tandori Boneless Chicken Thighs

Macros: Fat 68% | Protein 30% | Carbs 2%

Prep time:15 minutes | Cook time: 30 to 45 minutes | Serves 16

The flood of fat in chicken thighs is coming for you. We coat the thighs with great flavor of tandoori and the grilling will keep the thighs juicy. Without the bone, you can enjoy the chicken thighs entirely free.

- 2 (6-ounce / 170-g) containers plain Greek yogurt
- 2 tablespoons freshly grated ginger
- ½ teaspoon ground cloves
- 2 teaspoons kosher salt
- 1 teaspoon black pepper
- 4 teaspoons paprika
- 3 cloves garlic, minced
- 2 teaspoons ground cinnamon
- 2 teaspoons ground cumin
- 2 teaspoons ground coriander
- 16 chicken thighs
- 1 tablespoon olive oil

Mix together the yogurt, ginger, cloves, salt and pepper in a medium bowl. Add the paprika, garlic, cinnamon, cumin, and coriander. Stir well and set the marinade aside.

Rinse and pat dry the chicken thighs. Cut 4 to 5 slits in each thigh, then place in a plastic zip-top bag.

Pour the marinade over chicken, seal the bag and shake until it is coated completely. (Don't forget to press air out of it.). Put the bag in the refrigerator to marinate about 8 hours or overnight for the best results.

Preheat a grill to medium heat and lightly grease the grill grate with olive oil.

Get chicken out of the bag, and discard the marinade. Rub out the excess marinade with towel papers. Spray the chicken thighs with olive oil spray.

Grill the thighs about 2 minutes per side until nicely caramelized, then cook approximately 35 to 40 minutes until the internal temperature reaches at least 165°F (74°C) on an instant-read thermometer.

STORAGE: Store in an airtight container in the fridge for up to 4 days or in the freezer for up to 1 month.

REHEAT: Microwave, covered, until the desired temperature is reached or reheat in a frying pan or air fryer / instant pot, covered, on medium.

SERVE IT WITH: To make this a complete meal, it's best served with a whipped cucumber raita with plain Greek yogurt, crushed garlic, and a dash of salt.

PER SERVING

calories: 445 | fat: 33.8g | total carbs: 2.7g | fiber: 0.5g | protein: 32.9g

Lemon Herb Chicken Breasts

Macros: Fat 35% | Protein 63% | Carbs 2%

Prep time:10 minutes | Cook time: 25 to 30 minutes | Serves 2

If you're looking for an easy, simple, and drop-dead-delicious way to cook chicken breasts quickly, you've found it! It's guaranteed to win the hearts of friends and family!

- 2 skinless, boneless chicken breast halves
- 1 lemon, cut in half
- Salt and freshly ground black pepper, to taste
- 1 tablespoon extra virgin olive oil
- 1 pinch dried oregano
- 2 sprigs fresh parsley, for garnish

. Squeeze the juice from ½ lemon to a large bowl, then add the chicken breast, salt and pepper. Toss well.

. Meanwhile, heat the olive oil in a skillet over medium-low heat. Add the seasoned chicken breast, oregano, pepper, and juice from remaining lemon. Sauté for 6 to 10 minutes per side until the chicken is cooked through.

. Remove from the heat and garnish with fresh parsley.

STORAGE: Fried chicken left in the refrigerator is good only for 3 to 4 days.

REHEAT: To reheat, let it in the room temperature for an hour then place the chicken in an oven-safe dish, pour a cup of chicken broth in the bottom of the dish, and cover everything with foil. Place it in the oven, at 350°F (180°C), for about 25 minutes.

You can also set it on a plate covered and microwave it on medium for 2 to 5 minutes.

PER SERVING

calories: 337 | fat: 13.0g | total carbs: 2.0g | fiber: 0.3g | protein: 53.3g

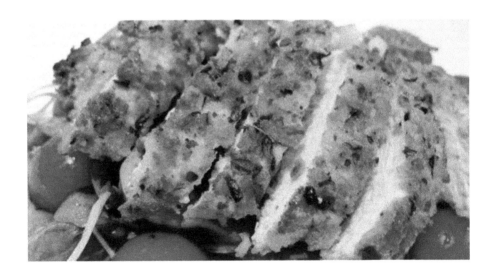

Lime Chicken Ginger

Macros: Fat 28% | Protein 66% | Carbs 6%

Prep time: 10 minutes | Cook time: 20 minutes | Serves 4

Chicken, a perfect meat to cook for any occasion. It's incredibly versatile and takes on flavors really well! Ginger and lime in the marinade used to produce this recipe create the ideal combination of flavors. The marinade can be made forwards and is easy to toss along with lime juice, lime zest, ginger, garlic, oil, sesame, and coriander.

And this lime chicken ginger is one meal that's perfect to make all year around. It is perfect to throw on the barbecue in the summer but is equally as good to grill in a pan and make a fresh salad or fajitas with any time of the year.

- 1½ pounds (680 g) boneless, skinless chicken breasts
- ¼ cup coconut aminos
- 2 tablespoons lime juice
- 2 teaspoons olive oil
- 1 teaspoon lime zest
- 1 teaspoon fresh ginger
- Pinch red pepper flakes, to taste
- 1 teaspoon sesame seeds, toasted
- 1 tablespoon fresh cilantro, chopped

Put the breasts of chicken in a huge, shallow dish. Poke holes in the chicken using a fork. This helps the chicken to drink the marinade.

Fill a small bowl with the aminos coconut, lime juice, olive oil, lime zest, ginger and red pepper flakes and blend to combine. Pour the mixture over the chicken and allow to marinate in the fridge for at least 3 hours.

Place over medium to high heat on a large grill pan. Once the pan is hot, add the chicken to the grill pan and pour the extra marinade over the top. Cook, turning halfway through until the chicken become golden brown and caramelized outside, and cooked for about 10 to 15 minutes all the way through.

Before eating, sprinkle with the red pepper flakes, sesame seeds and coriander.

STORAGE: Keeping foods separate and well covered helps to combat potential cross-contamination. store it in a plastic container in the fridge for up to 3 to 4 days or in the freezer for up to 3 weeks

REHEAT: Microwave, grill, covered, or reheated in frying pan or air fryer / instant pot. Don't reheat leftovers more than once. This is because the more times you cool and reheat food, the higher the risk of food poisoning.

SERVE IT WITH: Serve with salad or steamed low-carb vegetables.

PER SERVING

calories: 232 | fat: 7.2g | total carbs: 3.8g | fiber: 0.2g | protein: 38.5g

Roast Chicken With Broccoli And Garlic

Macros: Fat 68% | Protein 23% | Carbs 9%

Prep time: 10 minutes | Cook time: 45 minutes | Serves 4

Roast Chicken with broccoli and garlic -yum! It's a quick, savory, nutritious, cheap keto meal. Works well as a short dinner, or a balanced lunch box. It'll become a favorite go-to. Cooked chicken and broccoli in 45 minutes in a garlic butter sauce, all in one oven!

CHICKEN LEGS:

- 4 (5-ounce / 140-g) chicken legs
- 1 teaspoon garlic powder
- 2 tablespoons olive oil
- 1 tablespoon Italian seasoning
- ½ teaspoon salt (if not have salt in the Italian seasoning)
- Freshly ground black pepper, to taste

GARLIC BUTTER:

- 4 tablespoons unsalted butter, softened
- 2 garlic cloves, pressed
- 1 tablespoon fresh parsley, finely chopped
- Salt and freshly ground black pepper, to taste

BROCCOLI:

- 20 ounces (567 g) broccoli
- Salt, to taste

Preheat oven to 400°F (205°C).

Season both sides of chicken legs with salt, garlic powder, black pepper, and Italian seasoning.

Heat 1 tablespoon olive oil in a large skillet or cast iron pan over medium-high heat. Cook chicken breasts 4 to 5 minutes per side or until browned and cooked through and reaches 165°F (74°C).

Cut the broccoli into florets when the chicken is in the skillet, and slice   the stem. In a saucepan, boil in light salted water for 5 minutes. Drain and put the water on the lid to keep it warm.

In a bowl, mix all the ingredients for the garlic butter. And serve with chicken legs and broccoli.

STORAGE: store it in a glass or plastic container in the fridge for up to 3 to 4 days or in the freezer for up to 3 weeks.

REHEAT: Microwave, grill, covered, or reheated in frying pan or air fryer / instant pot. Don't reheat leftovers more than once.

SERVE IT WITH: Serve with broccoli and garlic butter on the chicken.

PER SERVING

calories: 494 | fat: 37.6g | total carbs: 12.1g | fiber: 4.1g | protein: 28.0g

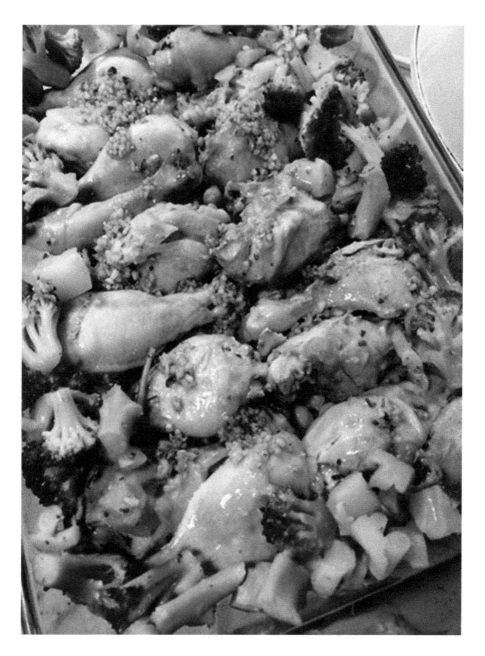

Mushrooms And Chicken With Tomato Cream

Macros: Fat 69% | Protein 24% | Carbs 7%

Prep time: 10 minutes | Cook time: 1 hour 30 minutes | Serves 4

This mushrooms and chicken with tomato cream is full of flavor and ready in less than 90 minutes. Elegant enough for a date night, fast enough and easy enough for a week-end dinner. It's sure to be a family favorite! I love this Chicken with Mushroom and Tomato cream! It's just so delicious. It is super- fast and simple

- 7 ounces (198 g) skinless, boneless chicken breasts
- 1 tablespoon olive oil
- Ground black pepper and sea salt, to taste
- 2 tablespoons salted butter
- 3 garlic cloves, minced
- 6 cremini mushrooms, thinly sliced
- 1 cup heavy whipping cream
- 3 ounces (85 g) Parmesan cheese, finely grated
- 4 ounces (113 g) fresh tomatoes, diced Fresh basil, for garnish

Season the chicken breasts generously with salt and pepper on both sides.

Heat up the olive oil over medium to high heat in a large skillet. Pan-sear the chicken breasts until each side is golden brown and caramelized, about 4 to 5 minutes. Take off the pan and cover to keep warm.

Add the butter, garlic and mushrooms to the same pan, reduce the heat to medium-low, and sauté until the garlic is fragrant and the mushrooms have released their liquid.

In the pan add the heavy cream, Parmesan and diced tomatoes. To thicken, mix in and let simmer, about 10 minutes.

Add the chicken back to the saucepan and cook until completely cooked.

Taste, and if necessary, add more salt and pepper.

Plate and top with fresh basil.

STORAGE: store it in a glass or plastic container in the fridge for up to 3 days or in the freezer for up to 2 weeks.

REHEAT: Microwave, grill, covered, or reheated in frying pan or air fryer / instant pot.

SERVE IT WITH: Serve with Loaded Cauliflower Salad.

PER SERVING

calories: 326 | fat: 25.6g | total carbs: 5.8g | fiber: 0.4g | protein: 18.5g

Simple Chicken Tonnato

Macros: Fat 71% | Protein 28% | Carbs 1%

Prep time: 10 minutes | Cook time: 20 minutes | Serves 4

Get your keto on with this amazing and simple chicken tonnato keto dish! Fall in love with fresh basil and rich tuna and enveloping savory chicken. It doesn't get much more keto-taste than this!

TONNATO SAUCE:

- 4 ounces (113 g) tuna
- 2 garlic cloves
- ¼ cup fresh basil, chopped
- 1 teaspoon dried parsley
- 2 tablespoons lemon juice
- ½ cup mayonnaise, keto-friendly
- ¼ cup olive oil
- ½ teaspoon salt
- ¼ teaspoon ground black pepper

CHICKEN:

- 1½ pounds (680g) chicken breasts
- Salt, to taste
- Water, as needed
- 7 ounces (198 g) leafy green

Mix all of the sauce ingredients in an immersion blender or in a food processor. Reserve the Tonnato sauce to allow the aromas to grow.

In a pot, put the chicken breasts with only enough lightly salted water to cover them. Bring to a boil.

Let simmer for around 15 minutes over medium heat, or until the chicken is completely cooked through. When you are using a meat thermometer, when finished, it will say 165 ☐ (74 ☐).

Enable the breasts of chicken to rest, at least 10 minutes before slicing.

Place the leafy greens on the serving plates, and top with the sliced chicken. Pour the sauce over the chicken and serve with a slice of fresh lemon and extra capers.

STORAGE: store it in a glass or plastic container in the fridge for up to 3 to 4 days or in the freezer for up to 1 month.

REHEAT: Grill, skillet, or reheated in frying pan or air fryer / instant pot.

SERVE IT WITH: Serve with beef stock and cauliflower rice.

PER SERVING

calories: 652 | fat: 51.3g | total carbs: 2.8g | fiber: 0.8g | protein: 43.2g

Chicken Nuggets With Fried Green Bean And Bbq-Mayo

Marcos: Fat 71% | Protein 24% | Carbs 5%

Prep time: 20 minutes | Cook time:25 minutes | Serves 6

Looking for another yummy scrummy keto meal? The Chicken nuggets with fried green bean is what you are looking for. As a young boy I used to eat nuggets all the time, and at that time I thought they were the best thing ever, so if you like normal nuggets as I do then surely these nuggets with BBQ-mayo and fried beans will blow your mind my friend. Chicken nuggets are not only for kids to enjoy, so make yourself this delicious meal and enjoy it regardless of your age.

There is no problem if you want to use chicken fingers instead of the nuggets.

CHICKEN NUGGETS:

- 1½ pounds (680 g) boneless chicken thighs, cut into bite size pieces
- 4 ounces (113 g) shredded Parmesan cheese
- 1 tablespoon onion powder
- ¼ tablespoon salt
- ¼ tablespoon ground black pepper
- 1 egg
- 1 tablespoon coconut oil

GREEN BEAN FRIES:

- 8ounces (227 g) fresh green beans, trimmed
- 1 tablespoon coconut oil
- ¾ cup mayonnaise, keto-friendly
- ½ tablespoon smoked chili powder
- 1 tablespoon garlic powder
- Salt and freshly ground black pepper, to taste

Put the Parmesan, onion powder, salt and pepper in a medium bowl and stir them till they are mixed very well

In another bowl, add the egg and whisk until it gets frothy.

Start Dipping the chicken pieces in the egg, and make sure to cover them entirely.

Coat the chicken nuggets in the Parmesan mixture by dipping them and shake off any excess.

Melt the coconut oil in a large skillet over medium heat, then fry the chicken nuggets on each side for 5 minutes until they become golden brown and cooked through.

Heat up coconut oil in a large skillet to medium-high, then put the trimmed beans and fry them for a couple of minutes. They should be crispy. Season the beans with salt before serving.

Now for the BBQ-mayo sauce, you should prepare a medium bowl and mix the mayonnaise, smoked chili powder, garlic powder, and a little bit of salt and pepper together, then stir very well and refrigerate for 30 minutes before serving.

STORAGE: Nuggets unfortunately last only for a day or two in the refrigerator. To maximize the quality of the nuggets. Wrap them with aluminum foil, or put them in a shallow airtight container.

REHEAT: It heats well in the microwave, but if you wanted them to be a bit tough then place the nuggets on a parchment paper lined cookie sheet, and make sure you preheat the oven to 350 □ (180°C), keeping them in there for 10 minutes will be enough to get them tasty and crunchy again.

SERVE IT WITH: There are a lot of things that could go along with this dish. Such as broccoli rice. The choices are not limited to certain things.

PER SERVING

calories: 644 | fat: 51.0g | total carbs: 8.5g | fiber: 1.7g | protein: 37.7g

MEAT

Hearty Calf's Liver Platter

Macros: Fat: 75% | Protein: 21% | Carbs: 4%

Prep time: 15 minutes | Cook time: 25 minutes | Serves 4

A wonderful liver and onions recipe makes a dinner. Caramelized onions enhance the flavor of liver in a delish way.

- ½ cup butter
- ¼ cup extra-virgin olive oil
- 2 onions, sliced thinly
- ½ cup dry white wine
- pound (454 g) calf's liver, trimmed and cut into strips
- 1 tablespoon balsamic vinegar
- tablespoons fresh parsley, chopped
- Sea salt and ground black pepper, to taste

In a large nonstick skillet, heat the butter and oil over medium heat until the butter melts. Sauté the onions for about 5 minutes. Stir in the white wine and immediately reduce the heat to medium-low. Cook covered for about 15 minutes, stirring occasionally. With a slotted spoon, transfer the onions to a plate.

Stir in the liver and vinegar and increase the heat to high. Cook for about 4 minutes more, stirring frequently. Add the cooked onions, parsley, salt and black pepper and stir to combine well.

Remove the liver mixture from heat and serve warm.

STORAGE: Store in an airtight container in the fridge for up to 4 days or in the freezer for up to 1 month.

REHEAT: Microwave, covered, until the desired temperature is reached or reheat in a frying pan or air fryer / instant pot, covered, on medium.

SERVE IT WITH: Broccoli mash is a great option to serve with this liver dish.

PER SERVING

calories: 497 | fat: 40.6g | total carbs: 7.9g | fiber: 3.0g | protein: 23.1g

Classic Sausage & Beef Meatloaf

Macros: Fat: 66% | Protein: 32% | Carbs: 2%

Prep time: 15 minutes | Cook time: 1 hour 15 minutes | Serves 6

A great-tasting baked feast of meatloaf for family and friend's dinner party! This meatloaf is flavored with the combo of ground beef, sausage meat, whipping cream, egg, veggies and herbs.

- 1½ pounds (680 g) Italian sausage, casing removed
- 1 pound (454 g) ground beef
- ½ cup almond flour
- 1 egg, beaten lightly
- ¼ cup heavy whipping cream
- ½ red bell pepper, seeded and chopped
- ½ of onion, chopped finely
- 2 teaspoons garlic, minced
- 1 teaspoon dried oregano, crushed
- ¼ teaspoon sea salt
- ⅛ teaspoon freshly ground black pepper

Preheat the oven to 400 □ (205°C).

Make the meatloaf: In a large bowl, place all ingredients and mix thoroughly until well combined.

Place the beef mixture into a loaf pan evenly and press lightly to smooth the top with your hands. Bake for about 1 hour to 1 hour 15 minutes, or until the internal temperature reaches 165 □ (74°C) on a meat thermometer.

Remove from the oven and drain off any grease. Let it cool for about 10 minutes before slicing to serve.

STORAGE: Store in an airtight container in the fridge for up to 4 days or in the freezer for about 1 month.

REHEAT: Microwave, covered, until the desired temperature is reached or reheat in a frying pan or air fryer / instant pot, covered, on medium.

SERVE IT WITH: This meatloaf goes well with mashed broccoli.

PER SERVING

calories: 479 | fat: 35.0g | total carbs: 4.0g | fiber: 1.5g | protein: 38.7g

Lemony Pork Loin Roast

Macros: Fat 38% | Protein 59% | Carbs 3%

Prep time: 5 minutes | Cook time: 30 minutes | Serves 10

This pork loin roast is known for its special marinade, which is made of onion with lemon juice, coconut aminos, garlic, and dried herbs. The roast is then dipped in this marinade for an hour, which enhances its taste and texture. Once cooked, the roast can be served with a range of low-carb veggies.

- ⅓ cup coconut aminos
- ½ cup lemon juice 1 red onion, sliced
- 1½ teaspoons garlic, chopped 1 tablespoon dried rosemary
- ¼ cup olive oil
- 1 (5-pound / 2.3-kg) boneless pork loin roast

Preheat the oven to 350 °F (180°C).

In a medium bowl, add coconut aminos, lemon juice, red onion slices, garlic, rosemary, and olive oil. Mix these ingredients well.

Pour this marinade into a Ziploc bag.

Place the pork loin roast in this bag and seal. Shake the bag well to coat the pork loin roast.

Transfer the roast and its marinade to a roasting pan and bake it for about 2 hours until the internal temperature of the pork reaches 165 □ (74°C).

Once roasted, remove the pork from the oven and allow to rest for 10 minutes. Slice and serve hot.

STORAGE: Store in a sealed airtight container in the fridge for up to 5 days or in your freezer for about 1 month.

REHEAT: Microwave, covered, until the desired temperature is reached or reheat in a frying pan or air fryer / instant pot, covered, on medium.

SERVE IT WITH: To add more flavors to this meal, serve the pork roast with crispy cauliflower pops. It also tastes great paired with sautéed spinach.

PER SERVING

calories: 346 | fat: 14.7g | total carbs: 2.7g | fiber: 0.1g | protein: 50.9g

Pork Chops Stuffed with Cheese-Bacon Mix

Macros: Fat 56% | Protein 43% | Carbs 1%

Prep time: 15 minutes | Cook time: 20 minutes | Serves 2

Now you can enjoy the pork loin chops with a rich and cheesy filling inside. The blue cheese is mixed with crispy bacon, chives, and basic seasonings, then filled in the pork chops pockets. You can add other varieties of cheese.

- 1 teaspoon olive oil
- 2 bacon slices, cooked and crumbled
- 2 tablespoons chopped fresh chives
- 4 ounces (113 g) crumbled blue cheese
- 2 boneless pork loin chops, butterflied
- Salt and freshly ground black pepper, to taste
- Freshly chopped parsley, for garnish

SPECIAL EQUIPMENT:

Toothpicks, soaked for at least 30 minutes

Preheat the oven to 325 □ (160°C). Lightly grease a shallow baking dish with olive oil and set aside.

In each pork loin chop, cut a slit about 2 inches deep and 3 inches long to form a pocket.

In a small bowl, add bacon, chives, and blue cheese. Stir well. Make two equal sized balls out of this mixture with your hands. Stuff each ball into the pork chop pockets.

Secure the edges of the chops with a toothpick and rub them with garlic salt and black pepper on the outside.

Arrange the stuffed chops in the greased baking dish and bake for 20 minutes in the preheated oven, or until a meat thermometer inserted into the thickest part of pork loin chops reaches 145°F (63°C).

Garnish with chopped parsley and serve warm.

STORAGE: Store in a sealed airtight container in the fridge for up to 2 days or in your freezer for about 1 month.

REHEAT: Microwave, covered, until the desired temperature is reached or reheat in a frying pan or air fryer / instant pot, covered, on medium.

SERVE IT WITH: To add more flavors to this meal, serve the pork chops with roasted cauliflower. It also tastes great paired with a tomato-cucumber salad.

PER SERVING

calories: 562 | fat: 35.1g | total carbs: 1.7g | fiber: 0.1g | protein: 57.0g

Oven-Baked Lamb Leg

Macros: Fat 67% | Protein 33% | Carbs 0%

Prep time: 15 minutes | Cook time: 2 hours | Serves 10

The time to serve the lamb leg is here! The roasted lamb leg is perfect servings for a large family, or you can serve it at a fancy festive dinner to treat your guests with its tempting aromas and flavors. By using just these 5 ingredients, you can cook yourself a complete low-carb meal.

- 5pounds (2.3 kg) leg of lamb
- 4 garlic cloves, sliced
- Salt and freshly ground black pepper, to taste
- 2 tablespoons fresh rosemary

Preheat the oven to 350 □ (180 □).

Using a sharp knife, cut several 3- to 4-inch slits in the top of the lamb leg, then stuff the garlic into the slits.

Sprinkle salt, black pepper over the leg and place it in a roasting pan.

Place the rosemary sprigs on top.

Roast the rosemary lamb for 2 hours in the preheated oven or until desired doneness.

Once roasted, leave the lamb at room temperature for 10 minutes before carving.

STORAGE: Store in a sealed airtight container in the fridge for up to 5 days or in your freezer for about 1 month.

REHEAT: Microwave, covered, until the desired temperature is reached or

reheat in a frying pan or air fryer / instant pot, covered, on medium.

SERVE IT WITH: To add more flavors to this meal, serve the lamb leg on top salad green. It also tastes great paired with a bowl of cucumber cream salad.

PER SERVING

calories: 524 | fat: 38.7g | total carbs: 0.5g | fiber: 0.1g | protein: 40.7g

Tangy Lamb Patties

Macros: Fat 60% | Protein 36% | Carbs 4%

Prep time: 10 minutes | Cook time: 15 minutes | Serves 4

This effortless lamb patties recipe can give you a hearty meal. You can cook these patties for dinner, or stuff them in low-carb buns or bread to make burgers or sandwiches, respectively.

- 3green onions, minced
- 1 pound (454 g) ground lamb 1 teaspoon ground cumin
- 4 garlic cloves, minced
- 1 tablespoon curry powder
- Salt and freshly ground black pepper, to taste
- ¼ teaspoon dried red pepper flakes 1 tablespoon olive oil

Preheat the grill to high heat.

Add green onion, lamb, cumin, garlic, curry powder, black pepper, red pepper flakes, and salt into a bowl, and mix them well.

Make 4 equal sized patties out of this mixture with your hands.

Lightly grease the grill grates with olive oil and grill the patties for 5 minutes per side until golden brown and slightly charred.

Let cool for 5 minutes before serving.

STORAGE: Store in a sealed airtight container in the fridge for up to 2 days or freeze the uncooked patties in your freezer for about 3 months.

REHEAT: Microwave, covered, until the desired temperature is reached or reheat in a frying pan or air fryer / instant pot, covered, on medium.

SERVE IT WITH: To add more flavors to this meal, serve the patties with tomato and avocado salad.

PER SERVING

calories: 264 | fat: 17.8g | total carbs: 3.0g | fiber: 1.3g | protein: 23.8g

FISH

Grilled White Fish with Zucchini and Kale Pesto

Macros: Fat 52% | Protein 39% | Carbs 9%

Prep time: 10 minutes | Cook time: 15 minutes | Serves 4

Would you like to brighten your dinner up, this is the best choice for you and your friends after a busy day. If you're a seafood person, you will love it.

KALE PESTO:

- 3 ounces (85 g) kale, chopped
- 1 garlic clove
- 3 tablespoons lemon juice
- 2 ounces (57 g) walnuts, shelled
- ½ teaspoon salt
- ¼ teaspoon ground black pepper
- 2 teaspoons olive oil

FISH AND ZUCCHINI:

- 2 zucchinis, rinsed and drained, cut into slices
- 2 tablespoons olive oil, divided
- Salt and freshly ground black pepper, to taste
- 1 teaspoon lemon juice

- 1½ pounds (680 g) white fish (such as cod), thawed at room temperature, if frozen

Make the kale pesto: Add the kale to the food processor with the garlic, lemon juice, and walnuts and blend, then sprinkle with salt and pepper for seasoning, and then add the olive oil and blend until the mixture becomes creamy and set aside until ready to serve.

Rub the zucchini slices with 1 tablespoon of olive oil, salt, pepper, and lemon juice and set aside.

Grease a nonstick skillet with remaining olive oil, and heat over medium- high heat.

Grill the fish in the skillet for 3 minutes on each side. Sprinkle with salt and black pepper, and serve with zucchini and kale pesto immediately.

STORAGE: We can store the leftovers in an airtight container in the freezer for up to 4 days. Pesto can be stored in the refrigerator for 3 to 4 days or in the freezer for up to 1 month.

REHEAT: Reheat the leftovers in the oven until warmed thoroughly.

SERVE IT WITH: To enjoy the meal, serve this dish with cauliflower rice and tangy cucumber salad.

PER SERVING

calories: 321 | fat: 19.5g | total carbs: 8.1g | fiber: 2.8g | protein: 30.3g

Cheesy Verde Shrimp

Macros: Fat 45% | Protein 50% | Carbs 5%

Prep time: 10 minutes | Cook time: 10 minutes | Serves 4

Ten minutes is all you need to create this delicious, healthy, and super tasty shrimp dish. These shrimps are thoroughly mixed with olive oil and garlic and topped with lots of Parmesan cheese.

- 2 tablespoons olive oil
- 2 garlic cloves, minced
- ¼ cup scallions, chopped
- 1 pound (454 g) fresh shrimps, deveined, and peeled
- ½ cup parsley, chopped
- ½ cup Parmesan cheese, grated

In a large skillet, heat the olive oil over medium heat.

Add the garlic and chopped scallions and sauté briefly, making sure the garlic does not turn brown.

Add the shrimps and cook until they become opaque. Sprinkle chopped parsley over the shrimp.

Remove cooked shrimps from heat. Serve on a dish and sprinkle with grated cheese.

STORAGE: Place the cooked shrimp in an airtight container and store in the fridge for up to 3 days.

REHEAT: Preheat the oven to 300 □ (150°C). Arrange shrimps in a single

layer on a cooking tray, and cover with aluminum foil. Place the covered tray in the oven and cook for around 15 minutes.

SERVE IT WITH: This dish goes well with warm kale salad, cauliflower rice, or zucchini noodles.

PER SERVING

calories: 215 | fat: 10.9g | total carbs: 3.2g | fiber: 0.4g | protein: 26.8g

Best Marinated Grilled Shrimp

Macros: Fat 47% | Protein 52% | Carbs 1%

Prep time:15 minutes | Cook time:6 minutes | Serves 6

A very simple and easy marinade that makes your shrimps so yummy and it doesn't even need any cocktail dressings. It's super easy, delicious and quick to make.

- ⅓ cup olive oil
- 3 cloves garlic, minced
- 2 tablespoons chopped fresh basil
- 2 tablespoons red wine vinegar
- ½ teaspoon salt
- ¼ teaspoon cayenne pepper
- 2 pounds (907 g) fresh shrimp, peeled and deveined
- 1 tablespoon olive oil, for greasing

SPECIAL EQUIPMENT:

6 wooden skewers, soaked for at least 30 minutes

Mix the olive oil, garlic, basil, red wine vinegar, salt, and cayenne in a large bowl. Stir in the shrimp and toss to coat well.

Cover the bowl with plastic wrap, then place in the refrigerator to marinate for 1 hour.

Preheat the grill to medium heat and lightly spray the grill grates with olive oil spray.

Thread the shrimp onto skewers, piercing once near the tail and once near the head, discarding the marinade.

Grill for 6 minutes, flipping occasionally, or until the shrimp is opaque.

Allow to cool for about 3 minutes and serve hot.

STORAGE: Store in an airtight container in the fridge for up to 3 days.

REHEAT: Microwave, covered, until the desired temperature is reached or reheat in a frying pan or air fryer / instant pot, covered, on medium.

SERVE IT WITH: To make this a complete meal, serve the shrimp with a glass of green smoothie.

PER SERVING

calories: 278 | fat: 14.6g | total carbs: 0.9g | fiber: 0.1g | protein: 36.4g

Salmon Fillets Baked with Dijon

Macros: Fat 40% | Protein 58% | Carbs 2%

Prep time: 10 minutes | Cook time: 15 minutes | Serves 4

Are you into seafood and want something fast, full of protein and keeping your keto routine? Salmon Fillets with Dijon is the one. A super rich dish that would be a true masterpiece on your table. Only in max 20 minutes.

- 4 (4-ounce / 113-g) salmon fillets
- ¼ cup butter, melted
- 3 tablespoons Dijon mustard
- Salt and freshly ground black pepper, to taste
- ⅛ cup coconut flour

Preheat the oven to 400°F (205°C) and line a baking pan with aluminum foil.

In a bowl, mix the salmon fillets, butter, mustard, salt and pepper. Stir well until the salmon is fully coated.

Place the salmon in the baking pan, then evenly sprinkle the coconut flour on top.

Transfer the pan into the preheated oven and bake until the salmon easily flakes when tested with a fork, about 15 minutes.

Remove from the oven and cool for 5 minutes before serving.

STORAGE: Store in an airtight container in the fridge for up to 3 to 4 days or in the freezer for up to 1 month.

REHEAT: Microwave, covered, until the desired temperature is reached or reheat in a frying pan or air fryer / instant pot, covered, on medium.

SERVE IT WITH: You can serve it alongside cauliflower rice.

PER SERVING

calories: 484 | fat: 21.6g | total carbs: 2.7g | fiber: 0.5g | protein: 70.1g

Salmon with Garlic Dijon Mustard

Macros: Fat 39% | Protein 57% | Carbs 4%

Prep time:15 minutes | Cook time: 20 minutes | Serves 4

Try this elegant salmon dish that is full of flavor. The mustard keeps the salmon moist and tender, and gives it an incredibly delicious taste!

- 1 tablespoon olive oil
- ⅓ cup Dijon mustard
- 4 (6-ounce / 170-g) salmon fillets
- 1 red onion, thinly sliced
- 4 large cloves garlic, thinly sliced
- Salt and freshly ground black pepper, to taste
- 1 teaspoon dried tarragon

Preheat the oven to 400°F (205°C) and grease a baking pan with olive oil.

Generously rub the Dijon mustard all over the salmon, then place the salmon in the pan, skin-side down.

Put the onion slices and garlic cloves on the salmon fillets. Sprinkle with salt, pepper, and tarragon.

Arrange the pan in the preheated oven and bake for 20 minutes, or until the salmon easily flakes when tested with a fork.

Remove from the heat and serve on a plate.

STORAGE: Store in an airtight container in the fridge for up to 2 days. Not recommend freezing.

REHEAT: Microwave the salmon and cucumber sauce, covered, until it reaches the desired temperature.

SERVE IT WITH: To make this a complete meal, you can serve it with rich chicken and mushroom broth and roasted asparagus.

PER SERVING

calories: 265 | fat: 11.6g | total carbs: 2.8g | fiber: 1.1g | protein: 36.0g

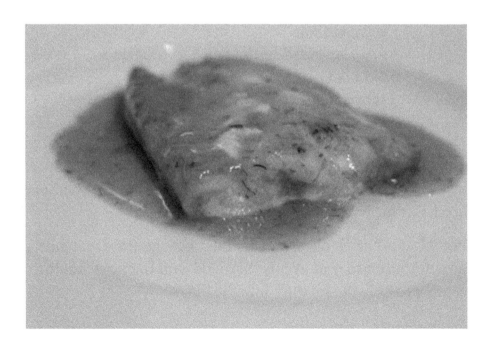

Blackened Trout

Macros: Fat 68% | Protein 31% | Carbs 1%

Prep time:20 minutes | Cook time: 10 minutes | Serves 6

Looking for an easy seafood dish that tastes great? Give this blackened trout recipe a try! The recipe calls for trout, but you can substitute for red snapper or catfish.

- 2 teaspoons dry mustard 1 tablespoon paprika
- 1 teaspoon ground cumin
- 1 teaspoon cayenne pepper
- 1 teaspoon white pepper
- 1 teaspoon black pepper
- 1 teaspoon dried thyme
- 1 teaspoon salt
- ¾ cup unsalted butter, melted 6 (4-ounce / 113-g) trout fillets
- 1 tablespoon olive oil

Combine the dry mustard, paprika, cumin, cayenne pepper, white pepper, black pepper, thyme, and salt in a medium bowl. Stir to combine and set aside.

Put ¾ cup butter on a platter, then dredge the trout fillets into the butter to coat evenly. Sprinkle with the spicy mixture, gently pressing the mixture into the fillets.

Heat the olive oil in a skillet over medium-high heat, then add the fillets. Cook the fish for about 2 to 3 minutes per side, turning occasionally, or until the fish is lightly browned on the edges.

Remove from the heat and serve warm.

STORAGE: Store in an airtight container and store in the fridge for 3 to 4 days or up to a month in the freezer.

REHEAT: Microwave, covered, until the desired temperature is reached or reheat in a frying pan or air fryer / instant pot, covered, on medium.

SERVE IT WITH: To make this a complete meal, you can serve it with beef stew, and kale and spinach salad.

PER SERVING

calories: 328| fat: 25.0g | total carbs: 1.7g | fiber: 0.8g | protein: 24.0g

Trout Fillets with Lemony Yogurt Sauce

Macros: Fat 36% | Protein 57% | Carbs 7%

Prep time: 12 minutes | Cook time: 8 to 10 minutes | Serves 4

Enjoy this tender trout that is served with a tangy, lemony yogurt sauce! This is definitely a recipe you will make several times for your family.

- 1 cup plain Greek yogurt
- 1 cucumber, shredded
- 1 teaspoon lemon zest
- 1 tablespoon extra-virgin olive oil
- Salt and freshly ground black pepper, to taste
- 2 tablespoons fresh dill weed, chopped
- 1 pinch lemon pepper
- 4 (6-ounce / 170-g) rainbow trout fillets

Mix the yogurt, cucumber, lemon zest, olive oil, salt, and pepper in a bowl. Stir thoroughly and set aside.

Preheat the oven to 400°F (205°C).

Sprinkle the lemon pepper on top and arrange the fillets in a greased baking dish.

Bake in the preheated oven for about 8 to 10 minutes or until fork-tender.

Remove from the oven and serve the fish alongside the yogurt sauce.

STORAGE: Store in an airtight container in the fridge for up to 2 days. Not recommend freezing.

REHEAT: Microwave the fillets, covered, until the desired temperature is reached.

SERVE IT WITH: To make this a complete meal, you can serve it with fresh cucumber soup.

PER SERVING

calories: 281 | fat: 11.4g | total carbs: 5.3g | fiber: 0.7g | protein: 37.6g

SOUPS

Sweet and Sour Chicken Soup with Celery

Macros: Fat: 37% | Protein: 57% | Carbs: 6%

Prep time: 5 minutes | Cook time: 30 minutes | Serves 10

This sweet and sour chicken soup dish is quick and easy to make and is perfect for busy weekdays. Made with delicious ingredients, this low-carb chicken soup is hearty and healthy and is perfect for all ages.

- 10 cups chicken broth
- 2 tablespoons butter
- 5 cups chicken, chopped and cooked
- ¼ cup apple cider
- 3 cups celery root, diced
- 1½ tablespoons curry powder
- 2 tablespoons Swerve
- ½ cup sour cream
- ¼ cup fresh parsley, chopped
- Salt and freshly ground black pepper to taste

In a large pot, mix the broth, butter, chicken, celery root, apple cider, and curry powder together. Let it boil for 30 minutes.

Fold in the Swerve, sour cream, parsley, salt, and pepper.

Serve into bowls while it is hot.

STORAGE: Store in an airtight container in the fridge for up to 4 days or in the freezer for up to 1 month.

REHEAT: Microwave, covered, until the desired temperature is reached or reheat in a frying pan or instant pot, covered, on medium.

SERVE IT WITH: To make this a complete meal, serve it with some parmesan roasted zucchini.

PER SERVING

calories: 178 | fat: 7.3g | total carbs: 3.6g | fiber: 1.1g | protein: 25.5g

Spicy Halibut in Tomato Soup

Macros: Fat: 32% | Protein: 58% | Carbs: 10%

Prep time: 5 minutes | Cook time: 30 minutes | Serves 10

This halibut in tomato soup dish is super easy to make and is a healthy fish soup. This delicious halibut soup is slow-cooked with garlic, tomatoes, and spices, which makes it a mouthwatering experience with every taste. It is a perfect dish for busy weekdays.

- 1 tablespoon olive oil
- 2 garlic cloves, minced
- ¼ cup fresh parsley, chopped
- 10 anchovies canned in oil, minced
- 1 teaspoon red chili flakes
- 6 cups vegetable broth
- 1 teaspoon black pepper
- 3 tomatoes, peeled and diced
- 1 teaspoon salt
- 1 pound (454 g) halibut fillets, chopped

In a large stockpot, heat the olive oil over medium heat. Add the garlic and half of the parsley and cook for 1 minute.

Mix in the anchovies, red chili flakes, vegetable broth, black pepper, tomatoes, and salt.

Reduce the heat to medium-low and let it cook for 20 minutes.

Put the halibut fillets into the pot and simmer for 10 minutes. Remove the halibut from the pot and put on a plate, then shred it with a fork.

Put the shredded fish back into the pot and let it cook for 2 minutes or until it is heated through.

Serve the soup with remaining parsley sprinkled on top.

STORAGE: Store in an airtight container in the fridge for up to 4 days or in the freezer for up to 1 month.

REHEAT: Microwave, covered, until the desired temperature is reached or reheat in a frying pan or instant pot, covered, on medium.

SERVE IT WITH: To make this a complete meal, serve it with some spinach salad.

PER SERVING

calories: 71 | fat: 2.5g | total carbs: 2.7g | fiber: 0.8g | protein: 10.2g

Spicy Shrimp and Chorizo Soup with Tomatoes and Avocado

Macros: Fat: 65% | Protein: 29% | Carbs: 6%

Prep time: 5 minutes | Cook time: 40 minutes | Serves 8

This Shrimp and chorizo soup packs the right amount of crunch and flavor with every spoonful. Made from the richest ingredients, it guarantees a fun family time and makes every experience a new journey.

- 2 tablespoons butter
- 3 medium celery stalks, diced
- 1 medium onion, diced
- 12 ounces (340 g) chorizo, diced
- 4 garlic cloves, sliced
- 1 teaspoon ground coriander
- 1½ teaspoons smoked paprika
- 1 teaspoon of sea salt
- 4 cups chicken broth
- 2 tomatoes, diced
- 1 pound (454 g) shrimp, peeled, deveined and chopped 2 tablespoons fresh cilantro, minced
- 1 avocado, diced
- Chopped fresh cilantro, for garnish

Heat half of the butter in a large pot over medium heat. Add the celery and onions to cook for 8 minutes.

Mix in the chorizo, garlic, coriander, half of the paprika, and salt, then let it cook for 1 minute.

Pour in the broth and the tomatoes and cook for 20 minutes and set aside

Heat the rest of the butter in a small pan over medium heat. Remove the chorizo from the broth and put it in the pan. Cook for 5 minutes until it is crispy.

Mix in the rest of the paprika and shrimp and let it cook for 4 minutes, then remove it from the heat and sprinkle with the cilantro.

Serve into bowls topped with the chorizo, avocado, and chopped cilantro.

STORAGE: Store in an airtight container in the fridge for up to 4 days or in the freezer for up to 1 month.

REHEAT: Microwave, covered, until the desired temperature is reached or reheat in a frying pan or instant pot, covered, on medium.

SERVE IT WITH: To make this a complete meal, serve it with a bowl of salad.

PER SERVING

calories: 325 | fat: 23.6g | total carbs: 7.2g | fiber: 2.7g | protein: 23.7g

Buttery Salmon and Leek Soup

Macros: Fat: 64% | Protein: 27% | Carbs: 9%

Prep time: 7 minutes | Cook time: 23 minutes | Serves 4

This buttery salmon and leek soup is a delicious low-carb dish for everyone. Packed with keto-friendly leeks, this creamy soup tastes like comfort with every bite. It is also quick and easy to make, which makes it perfect for busy weekdays.

- 2 tablespoons butter
- 2 leeks, rinsed, trimmed and sliced
- 3 garlic cloves, minced
- 6 cups seafood broth
- 2teaspoons dried thyme leaves
- Salt and freshly ground black pepper, to taste 1 pound (454 g) salmon, in bite-size pieces
- 1½ cups unsweetened coconut milk

Heat the butter in a pan over medium heat and add the leeks and garlic.

Cook for 3 minutes.

Mix in the broth and thyme to cook on low heat for 15 minutes, then season with salt and pepper.

Add the salmon and the coconut milk to the pot. Cook on low heat for 5 minutes.

Remove the pot from the heat and serve the soup into bowls while hot.

STORAGE: Store in an airtight container in the fridge for up to 4 days or in the freezer for up to 1 month.

REHEAT: Microwave, covered, until the desired temperature is reached or reheat in a frying pan or instant pot, covered, on medium.

SERVE IT WITH: To make this a complete meal, serve it with Parmesan roasted zucchini.

PER SERVING

calories: 506 | fat: 36.0g | total carbs: 13.9g | fiber: 3.0g | protein: 34.5g

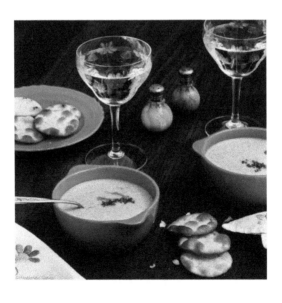

Sour and Spicy Shrimp Soup with Mushrooms

Macros: Fat: 45% | Protein: 41% | Carbs: 14%

Prep time: 10 minutes | Cook time: 39 minutes | Serves 6

This sour and spicy shrimp soup with mushrooms is a delicious dish laden with body-cleansing spices. This spicy soup can be a variety of things for anyone. From comfort food to a warm bowl, this shrimp soup brings seafood to your taste buds in unexplored ways.

- 3 tablespoons butter
- 1 pound (454 g) shrimp, peeled and deveined
- 1 piece ginger root, peeled
- ½ teaspoon fresh lime zest
- 1 medium onion, diced
- 4 garlic cloves
- 1 stalk lemongrass
- 1 red Thai chili, roughly chopped
- Salt and black pepper, to taste
- 5 cups chicken broth
- 1tablespoon coconut oil
- 1 small green zucchini
- ½ pound (227 g) cremini mushrooms, sliced into wedges
- 2 tablespoons fish sauce
- 2 tablespoons fresh lime juice
- ¼ cup fresh Thai basil, coarsely chopped

- ¼ bunch fresh cilantro, coarsely chopped

Heat the butter in a pot over medium heat and add the shrimps. Cook for 1 minute.

Mix it well with a wooden spoon and add the ginger root, lime zest, onion, garlic, lemongrass stalk, red Thai chili, salt, and pepper. Cook, covered, for 3 minutes.

. Pour the broth into the pot and let it cook for 30 minutes. Drain the liquid from the ingredients in the pot.

Put a pan over high heat and add the coconut oil, zucchini, and mushrooms to the pan, then season it with salt and pepper. Let fry for 3 minutes, then add the shrimp mixture.

Mix the contents of the pan and let it cook for 2 minutes, then add the fish sauce, lime juice, salt, and black pepper.

Let it cook for 1 minute and mix in the basil and cilantro.

Serve immediately.

STORAGE: Store in an airtight container in the fridge for up to 4 days or in the freezer for up to 1 month.

REHEAT: Microwave, covered, until the desired temperature is reached or reheat in a frying pan or instant pot, covered, on medium.

PER SERVING

calories: 180| fat: 9.1g | total carbs: 7.6g | fiber: 1.4g | protein: 18.4g

Creamy Garlic Pork with Cauliflower Soup

Macros: Fat: 68% | Protein: 21% | Carbs: 11%

Prep time: 10 minutes | Cook time: 39 minutes | Serves 6

This creamy garlic pork and cauliflower soup is the mouthwatering soup dish for all pork lovers. It is a low-carb alternative to having a creamy pork soup. It has a tangy taste from the garlic and the sour cream which would have you reaching for the next bite.

- ½ cup butter
- 1 medium onion
- 8 garlic cloves
- 1 pound (454 g) cauliflower
- 7 cups chicken broth
- 1 teaspoon of sea salt
- 2 teaspoons dried oregano
- 1½ cups pulled pork
- 3 tablespoons sour cream

SPECIAL EQUIPMENT:

Immersion blender

Heat the butter in a pan over medium heat and add the onions and garlic.

Cook for 3 minutes.

Add the cauliflower, broth, and salt and let it cook for 20 minutes. Remove it from the heat. Use an immersion blender to purée until it is smooth.

Mix in the oregano, then put it back on the heat and let it cook for 5 minutes.

Mix in the pork and the sour cream and let it cook for 15 minutes.

Serve into bowls, hot.

STORAGE: Store in an airtight container in the fridge for up to 4 days or in the freezer for up to 1 month.

REHEAT: Microwave, covered, until the desired temperature is reached or reheat in a frying pan or instant pot, covered, on medium.

SERVE IT WITH: To make this a complete meal, serve it with some spinach salad.

PER SERVING

calories: 247 | fat: 18.7g | total carbs: 8.9g | fiber: 2.0g | protein: 12.7g

Creamy Beef and Broccoli Soup

Macros: Fat: 59% | Protein: 26% | Carbs: 15%

Prep time: 4 minutes | Cook time: 46 minutes | Serves 6

The appeal of one-hour dishes cannot be overemphasized. This creamy beef and broccoli soup is the perfect soup for beef lovers. Made with an array of ingredients, the beef softly breaks down in your mouth while you enjoy the flavor-rich soup. This low-carb alternative helps cleanse the body while delivering great taste.

- 2 tablespoons avocado oil
- 1 onion, chopped
- 2 garlic cloves, minced
- 2 tablespoons Thai green curry paste
- 2-inch ginger, minced
- 1 Serrano pepper, minced
- 3 tablespoons coconut amino
- ½ teaspoon salt
- 1 pound (454 g) ground beef
- 2 teaspoons fish sauce
- ½ teaspoon black pepper
- 4 cups beef bone broth
- 1 cup unsweetened coconut milk
- 2 large broccoli stalks, cut into florets Cilantro, garnish

In a large pot, heat the oil and add the onions. Cook for 4 minutes then add the garlic, curry paste, ginger, and Serrano pepper to cook for 1 minute.

Add the coconut aminos, salt, ground beef, fish sauce, and black pepper and cook for 6 minutes.

Pour in the bone broth, then reduce the heat and cover the pot. Cook for 20 minutes.

Mix in the coconut milk and the broccoli florets. Cover the pot and cook for 10 minutes on high heat.

Reduce the heat and let it cook for another 5 minutes, then turn off the heat.

Serve the soup into bowls garnished with cilantro.

STORAGE: Store in an airtight container in the fridge for up to 4 days or in the freezer for up to 1 month.

REHEAT: Microwave, covered, until the desired temperature is reached or reheat in a frying pan or instant pot, covered, on medium.

SERVE IT WITH: To make this a complete meal, serve it with Parmesan roasted zucchini.

PER SERVING

calories: 424 | fat: 27.7g | total carbs: 18.0g | fiber: 1.4g | protein: 27.1g

Cheesy Sausage Soup with Tomatoes and Spinach

Macros: Fat: 69% | Protein: 22% | Carbs: 9%

Prep time: 2 minutes | Cook time: 6 hours 6 minutes | Serves 10

This delicious cheesy sausage soup is packed with delicious spices and ingredients, which makes it a perfect dish for everyone. Made with tomatoes and spinach, this soup bursts with a delicious flavor that delights your taste buds.

- 2 tablespoons extra virgin olive oil
- 2 pounds (907 g) hot Italian sausage cut into bite-size pieces 2 sweet bell peppers, chopped
- 2 cups chicken broth low sodium 4 garlic cloves, minced
- 1onion, chopped
- 2tablespoons red wine vinegar 2 cups of water
- 1 (28-ounce / 794-g) can diced tomatoes with juice 4 ounces (113 g) fresh spinach leaves
- 1 teaspoon dried basil
- 1teaspoon dried parsley
- ½ cup Parmesan cheese, grated

SPECIAL EQUIPMENT:

Slow cooker

Heat the olive oil in a pan over medium heat, then add the sausages. Cook for 5 minutes or until it is brown.

Put the cooked sausages into the slow cooker, then add the bell peppers, broth, garlic, onion, vinegar, water, and the tomatoes and its juice into the slow cooker. Cook on low for 6 hours.

Mix in the fresh spinach, basil, and parsley.

Serve into bowls topped with the grated Parmesan cheese.

STORAGE: Store in an airtight container in the fridge for up to 4 days or in the freezer for up to 1 month.

REHEAT: Microwave, covered, until the desired temperature is reached or reheat in a frying pan or instant pot, covered, on medium.

PER SERVING

calories: 387 | fat: 29.5g | total carbs: 11.9g | fiber: 2.9g | protein: 21.3g

SALADS & APPETIZERS

Chicken, Cranberry, and Pecan Salad

Macros: Fat 71% | Protein 21% | Carbs 8%

Prep time: 1 hour 10 minutes | Cook time: 0 minutes | Serves 12

It is a special salad made uniquely with ingredients that bring out a special fusion of flavor. It is a quick fix and a favorite among many people. The pecans and cranberry will send you the taste that comes from a different field of food.

- 1 teaspoon paprika
- 1 cup keto-friendly mayonnaise
- 1 teaspoon seasoning salt
- 1cup celery, chopped
- 1½ cups dried cranberries
- ½ cup green bell pepper, minced
- 1 cup chopped pecans
- 2 chopped green onions
- 4 cups cooked chicken meat, cubed
- Ground black pepper, to taste

In a medium bowl, add paprika, mayonnaise and seasoned salt. Stir well to mix.

Add the celery, dried cranberries, bell pepper, pecans and onion and stir well to combine. Add chicken cubes. Sprinkle with black pepper.

Let it rest in the refrigerator for 1 hour before serving.

STORAGE: Store in an airtight container in the refrigerator for up to 5 days.

SERVE IT WITH: To make this a complete meal, serve with beef and pork stuffed tomatoes.

PER SERVING

calories: 274 | fat: 21.7g | total carbs: 7.5g | fiber: 2.1g | protein: 14.2g

Crispy Almonds with Brussels Sprout Salad

Macros: Fat 84% | Protein 9% | Carbs 7%

Prep time: 12 minutes | Cook time: 10 minutes | Serves 4

It is a simple and fresh salad that is easy to prepare. The crispy and lemon touch brought about by the almonds and lemon makes it special. It is also very nutritious.

- 1 tablespoon coconut oil
- 1 teaspoon chili paste
- 2 ounces (57 g) almonds
- 1 ounce (28 g) pumpkin seeds
- ½ teaspoon fennel seeds
- 1 ounce (28 g) sunflower seeds
- 1 pinch salt

SALAD:

- 1 pound (454 g) Brussels sprouts, shredded
- 1 lemon, juice and zest
- ½ cup olive oil
- Salt and freshly ground black pepper, to taste
- ½ cup spicy almond and seed mix

In a frying pan, add oil and heat. Add chili, almond, pumpkin seeds, fennel seeds, and sunflower seeds into the oil and stir to mix.

Add salt and sauté for 2 minutes. Set aside until ready to serve.

Make the salad: Shred the Brussels sprouts in a food processor, then put in a bowl.

Combine the lemon juice and zest, olive oil, pepper and salt in a separate bowl, then pour the mixture over the Brussels sprouts. Toss to combine well and allow to marinate in the fridge for about 10 minutes.

On a serving plate, combine the salad and almond and seeds mixture before serving.

STORAGE: Store in an airtight container in the refrigerator for up to 4 days.

SERVE IT WITH: To make this a complete meal, serve with roasted salmon.

PER SERVING

calories: 484 | fat: 44.9g | total carbs: 16.8g | fiber: 7.9g | protein: 11.1g

Keto Lemon Dressing, Walnuts and Zucchini Salad

Macros: Fat 87% | Protein 4% | Carbs 9%

Prep time: 15 minutes | Cook time: 10 minutes | Serves 4

The salad is nutritious and low in carbohydrates. It is very easy to make and can serve with your friends and families. The walnuts contain abundant fat and is a very nice keto-friendly recipe, and it can be also eaten as the snack during the leisure time.

DRESSING:

- 2 teaspoons lemon juice
- 2 tablespoons olive oil
- 1 finely minced garlic clove
- ¾ cup keto-friendly mayonnaise
- ¼ teaspoon chili powder
- ½ teaspoon salt

SALAD:

- 4 ounces (113 g) arugula lettuce
- 1 head Romaine lettuce
- ¼ cup fresh chives, finely chopped
- 1 tablespoon olive oil
- 2 zucchinis, deseeded and cut into ½-inch pieces
- Salt and freshly ground black pepper, to taste
- 3½ ounces (99 g) toasted walnuts, chopped

Make the dressing: In a bowl, add lemon juice, olive oil, garlic, mayonnaise, chili powder and salt. Whisk together to mix and set aside.

Make the salad: In a large bowl, add arugula, Romaine, and chives and mix well. Set aside.

In a frying pan, add olive oil and heat over medium heat. Add zucchinis, pepper, salt, and sauté for 5 minutes or until the zucchinis are tender but still firm.

Transfer the zucchinis to the salad bowl, then add the toasted walnuts and pour over the dressing. Gently toss until fully combined. Serve immediately or refrigerate to chill.

STORAGE: Store in an airtight container in the refrigerator for up to 5 days.

SERVE IT WITH: To make this a complete meal, serve with grilled beef or shrimp skewers.

PER SERVING

calories: 587 | fat: 58.2g | total carbs: 13.9g | fiber: 6.7g | protein: 8.2g

Breaded Chicken Strips and Spinach Salad

Macros: Fat 73% | Protein 21% | Carbs 6%

Prep time: 15 minutes | Cook time: 25 minutes | Serves 4

Made with various flavors, you will enjoy the breaded chicken strips with fresh spinach salad for lunch or dinner. The meal has extra taste from coconut flavors that will leave you craving for more.

- 3 tablespoons refined avocado oil, for greasing the baking sheet

CHICKEN:

- 1 cup unsweetened shredded coconut
- 1 tablespoon plus
- 1 teaspoon Cajun seasoning
- 1½ pounds (680 g) boneless, skinless chicken thighs

SALAD:

- 4 cups fresh spinach
- ½ cup sliced green onions
- ½ cup roughly chopped celery
- 1 cup ranch dressing

Start by preheating the oven to 375 □ (190°C). Grease a baking sheet with the avocado oil generously and set aside.

Put the shredded coconut in a blender and pulse until grounded coarsely, but not to a powder.

In a medium bowl, put the shredded coconut and Cajun seasoning, then stir to mix thoroughly.

Using a mallet, pound the chicken thighs until it is ¼-inch thickness. Add the chicken to the bowl of coconut and Cajun seasoning. Toss until the chicken is coated well.

Arrange the chicken thighs on the greased baking sheet. Bake in the preheated oven for about 25 minutes, or until cooked through.

Meanwhile, make the salad: divide the spinach equally among four serving plates.

Sprinkle the green onions and celery on top.

Transfer the chicken to plates before slicing. Serve it with ranch dressing in a small bowl or ramekin on the side.

STORAGE: Store in a separate airtight container in the fridge for up to 3 days.

REHEAT: Microwave the chicken, covered, until the desired temperature is reached or put the chicken in a casserole dish then reheat in a preheated oven at 300 □ (150 □) until warmed through for 15 minutes.

PER SERVING

calories: 705 | fat: 56.7g | total carbs: 11.2g | fiber: 6.4g | protein: 37.6g

Veggies and Calamari Salad

Macros: Fat 54% | Protein 43% | Carbs 3%

Prep time: 10 minutes | Cook time: 7 minutes | Serves 4

Vegetable and calamari salad tastes perfect for lunch. If you have a group of friends visiting, this is a good recipe to surprise them with. Flavors from the lemon zest and lemon juice make the salad more delicious.

SALAD:

- 12 ounces (340 g) uncooked calamari rings
- 1½ cups grape halved tomatoes
- ½ cup kalamata olives, pitted and halved
- ½ packed cup fresh parsley, chopped
- ¼ cup sliced green onions

DRESSING:

- 1 tablespoon red wine vinegar
- ½ cup extra-virgin olive oil
- 2 small, minced garlic cloves
- ½ juiced lemon
- ½ grated lemon zest
- ¼ teaspoon black pepper
- ¼ teaspoon gray sea salt

Put the calamari in a steamer and steam for 7 minutes, then put in the freezer to cool for about 2 minutes.

In the meantime, start the dressing by putting all the dressing ingredients in a small bowl, then mix thoroughly and set aside.

Once the calamari has cooled, place it in a large bowl along with the   grape tomatoes, olives, parsley, and green onions. Pour in the dressing and toss to coat well.

Evenly divide the salad among four serving bowls and serve.

STORAGE: Store in an airtight container in the fridge for up to 3 days.

SERVE IT WITH: To make this a complete meal, you can serve it with rich clam chowder.

PER SERVING

calories: 508 | fat: 30g | total carbs: 4.4g | fiber: 1.3g | protein: 55.1g

Colorful Crab Ceviche Appetizer

Macros: Fat 37% | Protein 47% | Carbs 16%

Prep time: 40 minutes | Cook time: 0 minutes | Serves 4

Colorful crab ceviche appetizer is the best side meal when it comes to maintaining your keto routine. What's better than a fat-free, protein full meal? You can have it on any meal in the day. Best Latino meal!

- 1 (8-ounce / 227-g) package crab meat flakes
- 1 tablespoon olive oil
- ½ bundle cilantro, finely chopped
- 3 Serrano peppers, finely cut into small slices
- 2 large tomatoes, evenly chopped
- 1 red onion, finely chopped into slices
- ¼ cup lemon juice
- Salt and freshly ground black pepper, to taste

In a bowl, place the crab meat. Pour the olive oil slowly into the bowl of crab meat until well coated, then stir in the cilantro, Serrano peppers, tomato, and onion. Pour the lemon juice over the mixture and toss well.

Sprinkle with pepper and salt, then refrigerate for an hour before serving.

STORAGE: This appetizer can be stored in the fridge for no more than 2 days.

SERVE IT WITH: To make this a complete meal, serve it with roasted

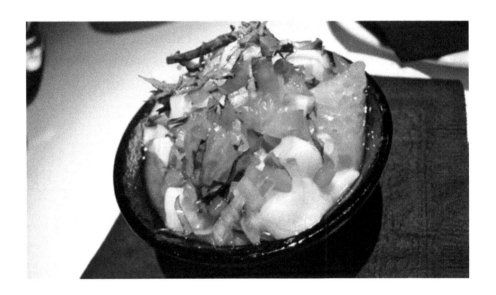

Mint and Tuna Salad

Macros: Fat 38% | Protein 54% | Carbs 8%

Prep time: 15 minutes | Cook time: 0 minutes | Serves 6

Did you know that mint is a rich source of vitamins A, C, B2 and valuable minerals such as calcium, copper and magnesium? Well, the Mint and Tuna Salad provide a magical combination of the fresh mint and the delicious tuna.

- 1 (5-ounce / 142-g) can tuna, drained
- 6 ounces (170 g) garlic and herb-flavored feta cheese, crumbled
- 3 hearts Romaine lettuce, cut into pieces
- 1 cucumber, peeled and chopped
- 4 green onions, chopped finely
- ¼ cup olive oil
- ¼ cup lemon juice
- 4 cloves garlic, diced finely
- ¼ cup fresh parsley, minced
- ¼ cup fresh mint leaves, minced
- Salt and freshly ground black pepper, to taste

In a bowl, mix together the tuna, feta cheese, lettuce, cucumber and green onion.

In another bowl, whisk together the olive oil, lemon juice, garlic, parsley, mint leaves, salt and pepper, then pour over the salad. Gently toss until well coated, then serve.

STORAGE: The salad can be stored covered in the fridge for 3 to 4 days.

SERVE IT WITH: The Mint and Tuna Salad can be a side dish with any other main dishes and will mix very well.

PER SERVING

calories: 418 | fat: 18.0g | total carbs: 9.5g | fiber: 1.5g | protein: 57.0g

Crab Salad

Macros: Fat 55% | Protein 42% | Carbs 3%

Prep time: 15 minutes | Cook time: 0 minutes | Serves 4

Love seafood and love to try the different seafood dishes? The Crab Salad is your choice for a simple but magically delicious meal. If you do not love to wait like me this salad would be just perfect.

- 2 pounds (907 g) crab meat
- 2½ cups celery, chopped finely
- ½ cup keto-friendly mayonnaise
- 2 teaspoons celery seed Paprika, to taste
- 4 teaspoons stevia
- ½ tablespoon freshly ground black pepper
- 1 teaspoon Old Bay Seasoning
- 2 teaspoons dried parsley

Mix the crab meat, chopped celery, mayonnaise, celery seed, paprika, stevia, pepper, Old Bay Seasoning and parsley in a large bowl. Stir with a fork to combine well.

Serve immediately or refrigerate to chill until ready to serve.

STORAGE: The salad can be stored covered in the fridge for 3 to 4 days.

SERVE IT WITH: To make this a complete meal, serve it with a bed of mixed salad greens.

PER SERVING

calories: 420 | fat: 26.1g | total carbs: 3.2g | fiber: 1.4g | protein: 41.7g

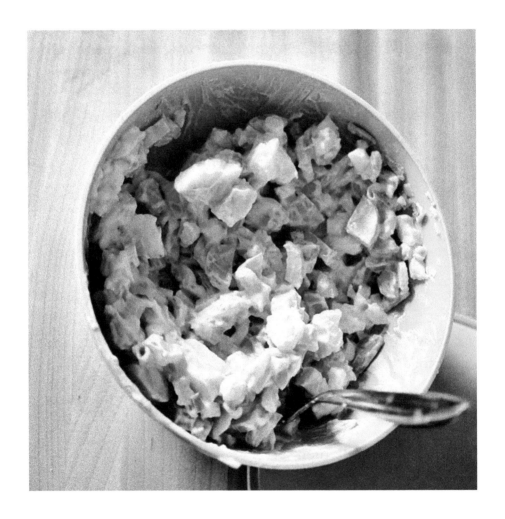

Tasty Shrimp Salad

Macros: Fat 71% | Protein 26% | Carbs 3%

Prep time: 15 minutes | Cook time: 0 minutes | Serves 6

This Tasty Shrimp Salad is one of my best ways to enjoy shrimp. It is so easy to do, and the results are amazing! The sea flavor of the shrimp and the freshness of eggs, cherry tomatoes, and celery will give you a perfect eating experience.

- 1 pound (454 g) cooked shrimp, peeled and deveined
- ¾ cup mayonnaise, keto-friendly
- 2hard-boiled eggs, chopped into chunks
- 1 cup cherry tomatoes, quartered
- Salt and freshly ground black pepper, to taste
- 1 cup celery, chopped
- ½ cup onion, chopped

In a bowl, mix the mayonnaise, eggs, tomatoes, salt, and pepper together.

Combine the mixture with the peeled shrimp. Add the celery and onion.

Toss to combine well, then serve.

STORAGE: The salad can be stored covered in the fridge for 3 to 4 days.

SERVE IT WITH: The shrimp salad can be a side dish with any other main dishes and will mix very well.

PER SERVING

calories: 322 | fat: 25.8g | total carbs: 2.8g | fiber: 0.7g | protein: 20.7g

Tuna Stuffed Avocados

Macros: Fat 64% | Protein 20% | Carbs 15%

Prep time: 20 minutes | Cook time: 0 minutes | Serves 4

Planning for a trip and needs something simple and freshening to take? Avocado and Tuna Tapas is the great mix you would consider for its perfect combination between avocado and tuna.

- 1 can (12-ounce / 340-g) solid white tuna, drained
- 1 tablespoon keto-friendly mayonnaise
- 3 cups thinly diced green onions, plus more for garnish
- ½ red bell pepper, chopped finely
- A dash of balsamic vinegar
- Garlic salt and ground black pepper, to taste
- 2 ripe avocados, pitted and cut in half

In a medium bowl, mix together tuna, mayonnaise, green onions, red bell pepper, and balsamic vinegar. Season with pepper and garlic salt. Using a spoon, stuff the avocado halves evenly with the tuna mixture.

Sprinkle the green onions on top for garnish before serving.

STORAGE: Store in an airtight container in the fridge for up to 3 days.

SERVE IT WITH: To make this a complete meal, serve it with roasted vegetables on the side.

PER SERVING

calories: 287 | fat: 21.5g | total carbs: 12.3g | fiber: 7.8g | protein: 14.4g

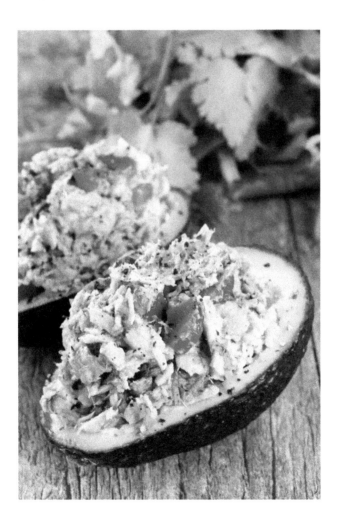

Chicken Salad with Ranch Dressing

Macros: Fat 76% | Protein 18% | Carbs 6%

Prep time: 5 minutes | Cook time: 20 minutes | Serve 4

Are you always looking for a delicious keto-friendly recipe? This chicken salad is low-carb and keto-friendly. It's healthy, easy and fresh.

RANCH DRESSING:

- 3 tablespoon keto-friendly mayonnaise
- 2 tablespoons water
- 1 tablespoon ranch seasoning
- 2 eggs
- 3 ounces (85 g) bacon
- ½ pound (227 g) rotisserie chicken, cut into smaller pieces
- 1 avocado, sliced
- 1 tomato, sliced
- 5 ounces (142 g) Romaine lettuce, chopped
- Salt and ground black pepper
- 2 ounces (57 g) blue cheese, crumbled
- 1 tablespoon fresh chives, minced

Make the ranch dressing: Combine the mayonnaise, water and ranch seasoning in a bowl. Set aside.

Boil the eggs in a pot of salted water for 10 minutes. Remove the eggs to a bowl of cold water. Peel and chop them into small chunks.

Fry bacon in a skillet over medium heat for 4 minutes per side until crispy. Remove from the heat to a paper towel-lined plate.

In a salad bowl, combine the bacon, chicken, sliced avocado and tomato, chopped eggs, and lettuce. Season with salt and pepper.

Drizzle with ranch dressing and top with blue cheese and chives before serving.

STORAGE: Store in an airtight container in the fridge for up to 3 days.

SERVE IT WITH: You can serve this dish with creamy chowder and fresh lemon juice.

PER SERVING

calories: 469 | fat: 37.9g | total carbs: 7.5g | fiber: 4.3g | protein: 26.8g

Caprese Salad

Macros: Fat 72% | Protein 25% | Carbs 3%

Prep time: 15 minutes | Cook time: 0 minutes | Serves 6

If you are a fan of salads as a side dish for your dinner, Caprese salad will be the greatest one as you do not need much effort or time to prepare it. With help from your children, you can make this splendid meal. In simple and easy steps, we will make it together!

- 1 pound (454 g) Mozzarella cheese, sliced into ¼ inch thick
- 4 large ripe tomatoes, cut into ¼-inch-thick slices
- ⅓ cup fresh basil leaves
- 3 tablespoons extra virgin olive oil
- Sea salt and freshly ground black pepper, to taste

Combine the sliced Mozzarella cheese, tomato slices, and basil leaves with a pinch of olive oil, sea salt, and pepper in a large bowl.

Leave the bowl in the refrigerator to chill for 20 minutes before serving.

STORAGE: Store in an airtight container in the fridge for up to 3 to 5 days.

SERVE IT WITH: To make this a complete meal, serve it chilled with pecan-crusted chicken nuggets.

PER SERVING

calories: 288 | fat: 23.8g | total carbs: 2.1g | fiber: 0.1g | protein: 16.9g

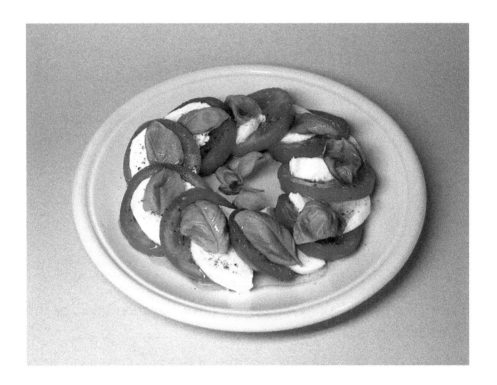

Baked Salsa Chicken

Macros: Fat 65% | Protein 31% | Carbs 4%

Prep time: 5 minutes | Cook time: 40 minutes | Serves 4

Do you wonder how to cook chicken in a healthy but surprisingly delicious way?

Baked Salsa Chicken will bring you a new way of perspective on salad.

- 1 tablespoon olive oil
- 4 skinless and boneless chicken breasts, halved
- 4 teaspoons mix taco seasoning
- 1 cup salsa
- 1 cup Cheddar cheese, shredded
- 2 tablespoons sour cream

Preheat the oven to 375°F (190°C).

Lightly grease a baking dish with olive oil, then arrange the chicken breasts on it.

Sprinkle with the mix taco seasoning and spread the salsa on top.

Bake in the preheated oven for 25 to 35minutes, or until the juices run clear.

Sprinkle the chicken with cheese evenly and continue baking for 3 to 5minutes more, or until the cheese is melted and bubbly. Top with sour cream to serve.

STORAGE: The dish can be wrapped with aluminum foil and stored in an airtight container in the fridge for up to 4 days or in the freezer for up to 1 month.

REHEAT: Microwave, covered, until the medium temperature is reached or reheat in a frying pan or air fryer / instant pot, covered, on medium.

SERVE IT WITH: You can serve it with leafy green salad or roasted vegetables on the side.

PER SERVING

calories: 508 | fat: 37.0g | total carbs: 5.6g | fiber: 0.5g | protein: 37.0g

Green Anchovy Dressing

Macros: Fat 99% | Protein 1% | Carbs 0%

Prep time: 10 minutes | Cook time: 5 minutes | Serves 6

Normal salad dressing is loaded with lots of sugar and processed chemical supplement and is forbidden to eat in keto diet. Well, creating a keto-friendly salad dressing becomes imminent! The green goddess dressing of 97% fat can be enjoyed contentedly pairing with your favorite vegetables without any worry.

- 1 green onion, chopped finely
- 2 cups keto-friendly mayonnaise
- 2 teaspoons fresh chives, chopped finely
- 4 anchovy fillets, minced
- 1 teaspoon fresh tarragon, chopped finely
- 1 tablespoon tarragon-flavored vinegar
- 2 teaspoons fresh parsley, chopped finely

In a bowl, mix together chopped green onion, mayonnaise, fresh chives, minced anchovy fillets, fresh tarragon, tarragon-flavored vinegar, and parsley until well combined.

Place the mixture in a jar and put it in the refrigerator for 20 minutes and serve chilled.

STORAGE: Stored in an airtight container in the refrigerator for about 1 week.

SERVE IT WITH: It can be served as a dip, or toss with salad greens for a dressing.

PER SERVING

calories: 555 | fat: 62.3g | total carbs: 0.5g | fiber: 0.1g | protein: 0.8g

Cheesy Keto Chicken Broccoli Casserole

Macros: Fat 74% | Protein 23% | Carbs 3%

Prep time: 15 minutes | Cook time: 35 minutes | Serves 6

The dish is an easy-and-quick side. You just need to prepare the ingredients and toss them in the oven for baking and move to busy work or entertainment activity. When the dish is done, the oven will call for you to enjoy the yummy meal!

- 2 tablespoons butter
- ¼ cup keto-friendly mayonnaise
- ½ cup Gouda cheese, shredded
- 8 ounces (227 g) softened cream cheese
- ¼ cup chicken broth
- 2 tablespoons dry ranch dressing mix
- 1¾ cups chicken, diced and well-cooked
- 2 cups cooked broccoli, cut into florets
- ½ teaspoon salt
- A pinch of ground black pepper
- 1½ cups Cheddar cheese, shredded

Preheat the oven to 350° F (180° C).

In a large nonstick skillet, melt the butter over medium heat. Mix in the mayonnaise, Gouda cheese, cream cheese, chicken broth and ranch dressing. Keep on stirring over low heat for 5 minutes until fully combined.

Add the chicken, broccoli, salt and pepper to the mixture. Stir well and transfer the mixture to a casserole dish, then sprinkle Cheddar cheese on the top.

Bake in the preheated oven for about 25 minutes. When the cheese is melted and the mixture is cooked, turn the oven to broil until the cheese gets browned.

Allow to cool for 5 minutes before serving.

STORAGE: Store the dish in an airtight container in the fridge for 3 days.

REHEAT: Microwave, covered, until the desired temperature is reached.

SERVE IT WITH: To make this a complete meal, you can serve it with roasted chicken thighs.

PER SERVING

calories: 541 | fat: 45.1g | total carbs: 4.9g | fiber: 0.8g | protein: 29.8g

EXTRA KETO TREATS

Keto Chocolate Coconut Candies

Yields Provided: 30 Servings

Macro Counts for Each Serving:

- Total Net Carbs: 0.9 g

- Fat Content: 7.8 g

- Protein: 1 g

- Calories: 78

List of Ingredients:

- Extra-virgin coconut oil (1 cup)

- Vanilla bean powder (1 tsp. or 1-2 vanilla beans)

- Raw cocoa powder (1 cup)

- Powdered erythritol/or your choice low-carb sweetener (.25 cup)

- Stevia extract (10-15 drops)

- Salt (1 pinch)

- Chilled Homemade Coconut & Pecan Butter - see below (.25 cup/2.2 oz.)

Preparation Technique:

1. Pour the oil into a small microwave-safe mixing container. Melt in the microwave using the low heat temperature setting for about a minute. Add the

erythritol, vanilla extract, stevia, and raw cocoa powder.

2. Mix well, removing all of the clumps.

3. Spoon the chocolate mixture into the silicone mold to about one-third of the way to the top. Place in the fridge until the chocolate solidifies (10-15 min.).

4. At that point, add .5 tsp. of the chilled coconut & pecan butter into the mold.

5. Top with the remaining chocolate mixture and pop it back in the fridge for at least 30 minutes to one hour or until firm.

6. Keep it refrigerated since coconut oil gets very soft at room temperature. Notes: Erythritol doesn't dissolve easily unless heated up. For a smoother texture, you can blend it until powdered.

Homemade Coconut & Pecan Butter

Macro Counts for Each Serving - 2 tbsp. each:

- Fat Content: 11.4 g

- Protein: 4.9 g

- Total Net Carbs: 2 g

- Calories: 151

List of Ingredients:

- Shredded - unsweetened coconut (2 cups)

- Pecan nuts (1 cup)

- Salt (.25-.5 tsp.)

- Sugar-free vanilla extract (1 tsp.) or (1-2 vanilla beans)

- Cinnamon (.5 tsp.)

Preparation Technique:

1. Slice the vanilla beans lengthwise to remove the seeds. Toss the pecans and shredded coconut into a food processor. Pulse until chopped.
2. Mix in the cinnamon and vanilla extract. Pulse all of the fixings until smooth for 30 to 60 seconds.
3. Empty the prepared butter into a glass container to cool at room temperature.
4. Notes: Toasting/baking the coconut & pecans for 5-8 minutes helps with the blending and enhances the flavor. Microwaving the butter for a few seconds will make it softer while refrigerating has the opposite effect.

Lemon Drop Gummies

Yields Provided: 4 Servings

Macro Counts for Each Serving:

- Total Net Carbs: 1 g

- Fat Content: 1 g

- Protein: 3 g

- Calories: 15

List of Ingredients:

- Fresh lemon juice (.25 cup)

- Water (1 tbsp.)

- Gelatin powder (2 tbsp.)

- Erythritol or stevia (2 tbsp.)

Preparation Technique:

1. In a small saucepan, heat up the lemon juice and water. Slowly stir in the gelatin powder and erythritol so that it all dissolves.
2. Empty into ice-cube trays or silicone molds.
3. Freeze or refrigerate for at least two hours.

Pecan Turtle Truffles

Yields Provided: 15 Servings

Macro Counts for Each Serving:

- Fat Content: 14 g

- Total Net Carbs: 1 g

- Protein: 4 g

- Calories: 142

List of Ingredients:

- Vanilla extract (.25 tsp.)

- Caramel extract (.5 tsp.)

- Swerve or your preference (.33 cup)

- Melted butter (.5 cup)

- Vanilla protein powder - zero carbs (.33 cup)

- Finely ground pecans (1 cup)

- Lindt or your choice - 85% chocolate (4 squares)

- Pecan halves (15)

Preparation Technique:

1. Mix the sweetener, butter, vanilla extract, caramel extracts, finely ground pecans and protein powder in a mixing container.
2. Roll into 15 truffles and place on a sheet of parchment or waxed paper.

3. Melt the chocolate in a baggie in the microwave for one minute. Snip the corner and squeeze the chocolate over the prepared truffles.
4. Garnish each truffle with a pecan half. Chill and enjoy any time.

Peppermint Bark

Yields Provided: 12 Servings

Macro Counts for Each Serving:

- Fat Content: 13.86 g

- Total Net Carbs: 1.89 g

- Protein: 0.47 g

- Calories: 131

List of Ingredients - Dark Chocolate Layer:

- Cocoa butter (.5 oz.)

- Peppermint extract (.5 tsp.)

- Lily's Dark Chocolate - chopped (4 oz.)

List of Ingredients - White Chocolate Layer

- Cocoa butter (2 oz.)

- Coconut oil (.25 cup)

- Powdered Swerve Sweetener (3 tbsp.)

- Peppermint extract (.5 tsp.)

List of Ingredients - Optional Garnish:

- Crushed peppermint candies (2 sugar-free)

Preparation Technique - Dark Chocolate Layer:

1. Mix the cocoa butter and chopped chocolate in a microwave-safe bowl. Using the high-temperature setting in 30-second increments, and stir until smooth. (Or, use the stovetop double-boiler style.)

2. Measure and add in the peppermint extract
3. If using silicone mini-muffin cups, use 12 larger muffin cups or 24 mini cups. Divide the chocolate between them. Pop the layer of chocolate into the freezer for at least half an hour to set.
4. Note: Option 2: Prepare the chocolate in an 8 by 8 pan with a layer of parchment paper.

Preparation Technique - White Chocolate Layer:

1. Melt the cocoa butter and coconut oil using the same process. Whisk in powdered sweetener and peppermint extract. Stir until smooth.
2. Empty the mixture into the chosen muffin cups or spread over the chocolate layer in the pan. Freeze for about 15- 20 minutes, until just starting to set, and sprinkle with crushed peppermint candies.
3. Place back into the freezer for an additional 30 minutes.

Strawberry Gummies

Yields Provided: 20 regular - 40 mini gummies

Macro Counts for Each Serving:

- Net Carbs: 0 g

- Fat Content: 0 g

- Protein: 0 g

- Calories: 3

List of Ingredients:

- Ripe organic strawberries (1 cup)

- Water (.75 cup)

- Premium Gelatin (2 tbsp.)

- Optional: Maple syrup (1 tsp.)

Preparation Technique:

1. Heat the water and berries in a pan on the stovetop until the mixture gets warm – not quite boiling. Remove from the burner.
2. Pour into a blender and mix sell. Empty the gelatin into the blender and mix again. Remove some of the froth. Let it sit for two to three minutes.
3. Mix lightly using a spatula. Pour into silicone molds of your choice.
4. Refrigerate for about four hours or until firm. Remove from the molds and serve to enjoy.

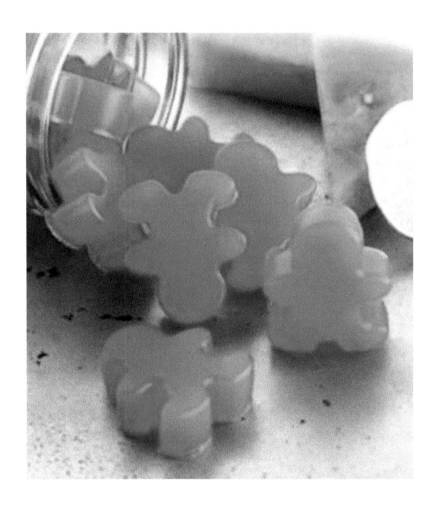